VENITA FREEMAN

The Practical Guide To Making Fitness A Daily Habit

Simple Ways to Improve Your Mental Health, Increase Your Lifespan, & Boost Your Immune System

This book was professionally typeset on Reedsy.
Find out more at reedsy.com

"In this trip around the sun we are only given one body. It is our job to take good care of it so it lasts for our entire ride on this planet!"

AUTHOR UNKNOWN

Contents

Introduction

Introduction

Have you ever started a new thing and stopped shortly after you started? Maybe you tried a diet, a fitness routine, or a treatment plan and gave up after a few weeks. Too often we wait until we get some kind of diagnosis to begin doing what we know we should have been doing already. We know that we should exercise at least 5 days per week but we often put that off or say that we don't have time for it. We also know that we should eat a healthy diet. We've heard about eating clean and we still choose foods that are fried, fatty, sugary, and the like. We know that portion size matters but we still order a large, extra large, or food for later, because the small one costs the same and we want to get our money's worth. We know that eating out is not the best for our bodies or our budgets but it's so convenient, so we continue. We know that we should sleep 7- 8 hours every night, yet we still don't make it a priority. We also know that drinking water is more beneficial to our bodies than any other beverage but there are so many other options that taste so much better.

We have a wealth of knowledge at our fingertips but we still choose options that will shorten our lifespan. What we need is a wealth of application. It's time for us to apply what we know and be consistent about it.We have to wake up before we end up with some life threatening or life altering illness.

Our lives are the sum total of all the decisions we make. Therefore we must be sure to set all excuses aside and choose to take action today and continue evermore.

Fitness goals are not reserved for the first two weeks in January. They are not only for acquiring our hot girl/boy summer body prior to going on vacation. Fitness is a lifestyle and should be a part of our daily experience. We simply decide that it is something that is important and valuable to us and make room for it. We are already good at making room for what's important to us (work, ministry, family, appetite, social media, phone calls, friends, shows, games, online accounts, portfolios, etc.). Let's make our physical bodies a part of our big picture. If we lose it, we can't use it. You matter. Your health matters. Choose to do better. Begin to apply what you know and start making some changes today.

1

Welcome

Welcome to your fitness journey! Incorporating daily exercise into your routine is not just about sculpting a toned physique; it's a key ingredient for overall well-being. Regular physical activity boosts energy levels, enhances mood, and improves sleep quality. It also plays a key role in maintaining a healthy weight, supporting heart health, and reducing the risk of chronic diseases. Besides the physical benefits, daily exercise helps your brain work better, making you think more clearly and make better decisions. It helps you deal with stress in a healthy way by releasing endorphins, which make you feel happier. Having a regular exercise routine makes you more disciplined, helps you recover faster, and boosts your mood, leading to personal growth in many areas of life. Let's experience this fitness adventure together while unlocking the benefits that daily exercise has to offer!

2

Top Priorities

Water

Drinking water is essential for several reasons. It helps maintain bodily functions, regulate body temperature, support digestion, and flush out toxins. Water is needed for nutrient absorption, joint lubrication, and overall cellular health. Staying hydrated also contributes to clearer skin, improves your ability to think clearly, and enhances energy levels.

The recommended amount is half your body weight in ounces. A person that weighs 200 pounds should be drinking 100 ounces of water. Drinking 8 - 8 oz glasses of water is not enough for everyone. It is too much for some and is not enough for others. Your urine color and fragrance is a great indicator of proper hydration for your body. It should be clear or lighter than lemonade.

Consuming enough water helps your blood flow, makes you feel full

so you can manage your weight, and prevents problems like headaches and constipation. It plays a key role in kidney function, helping to eliminate waste products from the body. Overall, drinking enough water is important for staying healthy and feeling good.

Managing Hunger

Warm drinks, especially low-calorie options like herbal tea (0 -5 calories/8 oz) and bone broths (30 - 50 calories/8 oz) can have a temporary impact on hunger. They may create a sensation of fullness, potentially reducing the immediate desire to eat. Additionally, warm beverages can have a soothing effect on the digestive system. However, the impact on hunger varies among individuals, and the effects are generally short-term. It's essential to consider overall dietary habits and nutritional needs for a balanced approach to managing hunger.

Sleep

Now let's talk about how our sleep keeps us fit. How we prioritize our sleep is important. Eight hours is still the recommended amount for most adults. A select few with a special gene can get by on 6-7 hours regularly. Getting enough sleep is crucial for various reasons. It supports our overall well-being, enhances cognitive function, boosts the immune system, and contributes to better emotional and mental health. Adequate sleep also plays a role in maintaining a healthy weight and promoting physical recovery.

Not only is the quantity of sleep important but consistency in our sleep schedule is also a key part of our well being. Did you know that it takes

4 days on average for our body to recover from deviations in our sleep schedule? A person who normally goes to bed at 10:00 pm during the week, should keep that same schedule every day of the week. Of course, there will be exceptions from time to time. If we're not getting enough sleep or our sleep schedule is inconsistent, then that's a great area to target.

It's time for us to consistently apply what we know about health and fitness. There are so many benefits for being active physically. We just have to find what works for us and continue doing it each day. Keep reading to find out how beneficial daily fitness is.

TOP PRIORITIES

3

Several Benefits

Physical Health Benefits

Regular exercise benefits cardiovascular health by strengthening the heart, improving blood circulation, and lowering blood pressure. It enhances the efficiency of your heart, allowing it to pump blood more effectively. Additionally, exercise helps reduce LDL (bad) cholesterol levels, while increasing HDL (good) cholesterol, promoting overall heart health and reducing the risk of cardiovascular diseases.

Furthermore, consistent physical activity contributes to maintaining a healthy weight and reducing excess body fat, which are crucial factors in preventing heart-related issues. Exercise also enhances the body's ability to manage stress and improves sleep quality, both of which play significant roles in cardiovascular well-being. Engaging in aerobic exercises like running, swimming, or cycling specifically targets cardiovascular fitness, making the heart and lungs more resilient over time.

Moreover, regular exercise promotes the dilation of blood vessels, improving their flexibility and reducing the risk of plaque buildup. It positively influences the body's insulin sensitivity, aiding in better blood sugar control and reducing the likelihood of developing diabetes, a condition closely linked to cardiovascular problems. The cumulative effect of these benefits creates a strong foundation for a healthier cardiovascular system, enhancing overall quality of life

Regular exercise also enhances muscle strength by causing microscopic damage to muscle fibers during workouts. As the body repairs these fibers, they become thicker and stronger, leading to improved overall muscle strength. Additionally, exercises such as resistance training and weightlifting stimulate muscle growth and development.

Three examples of resistance training exercises are push-ups, dumbbell bicep curls, and squats.

1. Push-ups: This exercise strengthens the chest, shoulders, and arms by using your body weight as resistance against gravity.
2. Dumbbell Bicep Curls: Holding dumbbells in each hand, you curl the weights towards your shoulders, targeting the biceps muscles.
3. Squats: Squats work the lower body, including the quadriceps, hamstrings, and glutes, by squatting down and standing back up while holding a barbell or using body weight as resistance.

Also, consistent physical activity enhances flexibility by increasing the range of motion in joints. Stretching exercises promote flexibility by lengthening muscles and improving their elasticity. This, in turn, reduces the risk of injury, improves posture, and allows for better coordination and balance during activities. like lifting weights, and flexibility exercises, like stretching, helps your muscles and bones stay strong and able to move well.

Also, exercising regularly helps make collagen, a protein that keeps tendons and ligaments flexible and stretchy. It also brings more blood to muscles, giving them the nutrients and oxygen they need to heal and work well.

Engaging in activities like yoga or Pilates specifically targets flexibility and balance, helping to maintain joint health and prevent stiffness. The combination of strength and flexibility not only improves athletic performance but also enhances daily activities and reduces the risk of injuries. Consistency is key in building and maintaining both muscle strength and flexibility.

Mental Health Benefits

Did you know that regular exercise is like a superhero for your stress levels and mood. Exercise helps our brains stay healthy and strong, just like it helps our muscles. It increases blood flow to the brain, which helps grow new brain cells and makes it easier for your brain to learn and remember things. Exercise also helps lower inflammation and stress in the brain. So, it's basically a stress-busting, mood-boosting dual impact device. Exercise is a known way to improve mental health by reducing symptoms of anxiety and depression. A brisk walk, a dance party in your living room, or even some yoga in your PJs can do the trick. So, get moving and imagine your stress melting away while you're breaking a sweat – it's like a therapy session, but with dumbbells and running shoes.

Daily fitness also has a positive impact on your sleep. When you work up a sweat during the day, your body temperature rises, and as you cool down post-exercise, it triggers a natural drop in temperature that signals to your body, "Hey, it's time for some shut-eye!" Exercise kicks stress to the curb, releasing those feel-good endorphins that act like a lullaby for your mind. It's like your body saying, "Thanks for the workout, now let's recline and recharge for tomorrow!"

Long-term Health Benefits

Exercising often is really important for staying healthy and stopping long-lasting illnesses. It helps your heart, keeps your blood sugar steady, lowers swelling, and helps you stay at a good weight. It lowers the risk of conditions such as heart disease, type 2 diabetes, and certain cancers. Doing exercise regularly helps you live longer and healthier because it makes your body and mind feel better in many ways. Another good thing about exercising every day is that it makes your bones stronger and keeps your joints healthy. It helps your bones grow, stops them from getting weaker, and keeps your joints flexible and strong. Regular weight-bearing exercises, such as walking and strength training, help prevent osteoporosis and reduce the risk of fractures and joint-related issues. Overall, daily fitness positively impacts life expectancy by reducing the risk of chronic diseases, enhancing cardiovascular health, and promoting overall physical and mental well-being.

Boosted Immune System

Regular exercise can strengthen the immune system by promoting good circulation. Good circulation allows immune cells to move more freely and do their job effectively, while also reducing inflammation and stress hormones that can weaken the immune response.

Social & Emotional Benefits

Group fitness activities, like playing soccer or joining a dance class, help people feel like they belong to a team. When you participate in group fitness activities, you not only get to have fun, but you also build a sense of community. Working out with others means you can cheer each other on and celebrate everyone's progress. This teamwork makes everyone feel important and included. When you know others are supporting you, it is easier to stay motivated.

Also, when you exercise, your body gets stronger and healthier, which makes you feel good about yourself. As you get better at the activities, your confidence grows, and you believe more in your abilities. This boost in self-esteem helps you feel happier and more positive every day. This boost in your self-esteem makes you more confident in other parts of your life, too. So, group fitness is great for both your body and your mind!

4

What To Do

Get Started

Small changes over long periods of time make big impacts. Pick an area of your life and start making small changes there. If you know that you are a couch potato and that chips are your thing, then do something about one of those things first. Do something about the chips or do something about your movement. If you continue to consume more calories than you burn then your body will continue to expand. If your body isn't expanding then it is simply becoming more toxic in a smaller space and those toxins are more likely to start affecting your vital organs.

A small step to take in this instance is to replace the chips you're eating with a baked chip or a natural chip. Perhaps you already eat baked or natural chips but you let yourself eat the entire bag. Try to reduce your consumption to a few handfuls and eventually graduate to the serving size that is recommended on the back of the bag.

Most of the time that we are sitting on the couch we are usually watching something. I know that some of us pay extra to not have commercials and ads during our shows. It's time to get up. Move the couch away from the wall and do some laps around the furniture while the commercials are going. If your show does not have ads or commercials, you can set a timer for 3-5 minutes and walk around the furniture before and after your show. This may seem odd but it's ok to be different. If you want something you've never had, you must be willing to do things you've never done. Movement helps burn calories. Choose something that will work for you. If you like going to the gym then do that. If you are at the store often, then park far away and visit a few locations or several sections in the store. If you are at home a lot, then jog in place, walk around the neighborhood, or find a YouTube fitness video that suits you. There are many 5, 7, and 10 minute videos that are easy to implement. The gym is not for everyone but movement is. Find something that will work for you and be consistent with it. You have the rest of your life to make it work for you.

Consistency With Accountability

One way to be consistent is with an accountability partner. If you know that you need to get in the bed earlier, drink more water, or eat more vegetables, then you qualify for an accountability partner. If you are on social media way too often, binge watch a lot of shows, or play phone, console, or computer games too much, an accountability partner can help you make gradual progress towards balancing that out. Find someone that is encouraging and set a day and time to check in with that person. If one day is not enough then you may need an additional partner or a second check in time. The check in time can happen in any way. You can choose a time when you will see that person face to face. You can do Facetime, Zoom, or a regular phone call. If brevity is your thing because life is busy, then you can simply give an update via text. For any commitment that you have, you are more likely to achieve it when you have someone that is encouraging you along the way and reminding you of your reason for doing it. Begin to tackle some of your desired achievements by finding someone that will hold you accountable to sticking to your commitments. This can also come in the form of a life coach.

Life Coach

Working with a life coach can offer many benefits. Below are three key advantages:

1. Clarity and Goal Setting: A life coach helps individuals gain clarity about their goals, values, and purpose. They assist in identifying what truly matters to the person and in setting specific, achievable goals. This structured approach can lead to a more focused and motivated pursuit of personal and professional aspirations.

2. Accountability and Motivation: Life coaches provide a level of accountability that is often difficult to achieve alone. Regular sessions with a coach ensure that individuals stay on track with their goals, maintain momentum, and are held accountable for their progress. This support can significantly boost motivation and drive.

3. Personal Development and Growth: Through guidance, feedback, and constructive criticism, life coaches help individuals develop self-awareness, improve skills, and overcome limiting beliefs. This process fosters personal growth and equips individuals with the tools and

strategies needed to handle challenges and achieve long-term success.

Life coaches usually charge for their services but are a great resource.

De-Stressing/ Body Balance/ Self Regulation Tips

- **4 Corner Deep Breathing**

1. *Find an object nearby that has four corners—a box, your monitor, or even this page.*
2. *Start at the upper-left-hand corner and inhale for four counts. Breathe in, filling your lungs with air.*
3. *Turn your gaze to the upper-right-hand corner and hold your breath for four counts.*
4. *Move to the lower-right-hand corner. Exhale for four counts.*
5. *Now shift your attention to the lower-left-hand corner. Tell yourself to relax and smile.*

Repeat these steps 3 to 5 times, or as often as you like.

- **ICE:** Inhale, Count **to 5,** Exhale

Feel free to count to 10 or 15 if that's what your body needs.

- **Roses & Candles:** pretend to smell roses and blow out candles **(3-5 repetitions)**

- **1 Minute Jog & a Stretch:** Set a 1 minute timer and jog in place. Then stretch: head up, head down, ear on your shoulder, ear on your other shoulder, roll your shoulders forward, roll your shoulders backwards, flamingoes, toe touch, side lunge to the left and right

- **Selfie Hug:** Put your arms straight out in front of you, cross them at the wrists, turn them so that your thumbs are facing downward to make the palms go together, interlock your fingers, tuck the interlocked fingers downward and let them rest under your chin while your elbows rest on your chest, then squeeze like you are giving yourself a big hug for a count of 10. Release and shake out your upper body. Repeat if desired

- **Alternating Nostril Breathing:** Sit in a comfortable, upright position with your spine straight. Close your eyes and relax your shoulders. Lightly rest your pointer and index finger between your eyebrows. Place your left hand on your left knee. Use your right hand to control your nostrils. Use your thumb to close the right nostril and your ring finger to close the left nostril. Gently press your right thumb against your right nostril to close it. Inhale slowly and deeply through your left nostril. After the inhalation, close your left nostril with your ring finger. Release your right nostril and exhale slowly and completely through your right nostril. Inhale slowly and deeply through your right nostril. Repeat until you are calm and relaxed.

5

Making Fitness Fit

Plan Your Work

Decide which activities you want to do and when you want to do them.

Work Your Plan

Dedicate 5 - 10 minutes or more each day to meeting your fitness needs by blocking it off on your calendar and by setting an alarm or reminder. The alarm and reminder are tools to remind you to get started. Another one can be set to remind you to end too.

Even though the ideal time is 30 minutes per day, 5 - 10 is an amount that is more reasonable for even the busiest of people. It is a great starting point and definitely can fit into your daily schedule. You can increase it at any point.

If you want to make fitness fit into your daily life, you have to say no to the millions of excuses that will come. Wake up with a YES on your mind and go with it. The easiest way to start is to stay in bed and ride your pretend bike or do a few stretches before you get up. There are a ton of great ab workouts that you can do while in bed. A few minutes of exercise first thing in the morning will get your day off to a good start instead of a groggy one.

Another simple thing that you can do is stretch, walk, or jog/march in place as soon as you get out of the bed. Start with 5-10 minutes and continue with that until you are doing it daily. There are several YouTube videos that offer short walks, stretches, and full body workouts. Find some that you like and go for it. You surely can find someone on YouTube that is doing fitness at a level you are comfortable with and one that fits your stage of life. The videos are set to all kinds of music and time periods. Be sure to include particular details in your search, i.e., 10 minute fitness to upbeat/classical/popular songs; 5 minute stretches to instrumental music, or 2,000 steps in 10 minutes, etc. Once you know the routine, you can silence the music that goes with the video and play your own.

Another way to get fitness in is to do it wherever you are. If your first need is a trip to the restroom, you can march in place there while you brush your teeth and comb your hair.

You can do 3-5 minutes of standing and sitting too. While your coffee is brewing, you can step out to the backyard or pause right in the kitchen and jump rope for that short time. A pretend rope works just as well as a real one. Consider your ceiling height and surroundings if you plan to use the real rope indoors. The goal is to get started and be consistent. Only ask yourself, "How can I make this work for me?".

Additionally, if you are working or shopping at brick and mortar places, you can choose to park far. This allows you to get a few hundred - 1,000 more steps. You can also do a lap or two around the inside or outside of the building as well.

6

Apps

We have so many apps to choose from these days. Most of the fitness ones come with a free trial period. Then you have to make a decision about continuing with the service. There is something for everyone. Noom and Just Fit are two apps that millions of people are using.

As of 2024, Noom has approximately 3.7 million active subscribers and remains a leading player due to its personalized approach to weight management and behavior change. The app has been downloaded over 45 million times across more than 100 countries.

Noom also assigns a coach to each subscriber. If you have questions or challenges that you need to talk through, your coach is your best cheerleader. They are great at keeping you encouraged and being a listening ear but are not licensed therapists.

Noom Mood is not as widely talked about but is just as valuable as the fitness version. It is geared toward helping people reduce their stress and develop the skills to manage it effectively. Noom Mood is a great fit for anyone that is interested in managing their stress and mental well being. It helps with reaching mental/emotional fitness milestones and will equip you with strategies and techniques for reducing stress and becoming more emotionally aware and resilient.

Let 's talk a little about Just Fit. As of 2024, the JustFit app has more than 2.5 million users worldwide. This app offers a variety of workout programs tailored to individual fitness levels and goals, including lazy workouts that require minimal equipment and effort. Just fit lets you choose exercises that are right for your age, ailments, limitations, and attitude. You may still need to modify some, but most of them will be just right.

7

Compounding Time

Another way to take charge is by compounding time while doing daily tasks. Incorporating movement into daily tasks can enhance physical health and productivity. Here are four ways to do this:

- **Walking Meetings/Meetups:** Instead of sitting in a conference room or at a desk, hold meetings while walking. Meet up with a friend for a walk and talk at a park or a mall instead of a restaurant. This not only promotes physical activity but can also stimulate creativity and engagement, and promote financial responsibility.

- **Active Commuting:** Choose to walk or bike to work or other regular destinations instead of driving or using public transport. If this isn't possible for the entire distance, consider parking further away or arriving early to walk a lap or two around the interior or exterior of the building. Also getting off public transport a few stops early is another option.

- **Desk Exercises:** Integrate simple exercises into your work routine, such as standing up to stretch, doing calf raises or marching in place while on phone calls, or using a stability ball as a chair. This can help reduce the negative effects of prolonged sitting.

- **Fueling Up Fitness:** While pumping gas, walk laps around your vehicle. Turn your music up and start walking. It's that simple.

8

Habit Bundling

Habit Bundling is also pretty popular. With this, you are pairing a behavior you want to develop with one you already enjoy. This method combines a desired habit with an established routine to make positive behaviors more permanent. You're more likely to continue with a behavior when you are doing it with one of your favorite things at the same time.

Bundled Stationary Exercises:

- Only visit social media while marching in place.
- Only listen to podcasts while doing arm circles.
- Only watch your favorite shows while doing seated leg lifts.
- Only talk on the phone while doing calf raises.
- Only eat at your favorite restaurant once you have exercised 4 or more consecutive days during the week.

Identify the things that you love to do or normally do and couple them with simple exercises like leg lifts, chair sits, and stomach vacuums. These stationary exercises are effective for improving strength, flexibility, and cardiovascular health without the need for much space or specialized equipment.

More Stationary Exercises:

- **Body Weight Exercises:** Squats, lunges, push-ups, and planks can be done without moving from one spot.
- **Isometric Exercises:** Holding a position, like a wall sit or a plank, helps build strength and requires minimal movement.
- **Jumping Jacks:** A simple cardio exercise that requires minimal space.
- **High Knees:** Running or walking in place by lifting your knees high engages the muscles and raises your heart rate.
- **Chair Dips:** Using a sturdy chair for tricep dips to work on arm strength.
- **Calf Raises:** Stand on a flat surface and lift your heels off the ground, engaging your calf muscles.
- **Seated Leg Lifts:** Sit on a chair or the floor and lift your legs straight out in front of you to target the core and leg muscles.
- **Leg Circles:** While lying on your back, lift one leg and make circular motions in the air. Switch legs after a set.
- **Arm Circles:** Extend your arms to the sides and make circular motions, both clockwise and counterclockwise, to engage shoulder muscles.
- **Stomach Vacuums:** Exhale completely, then suck in your stomach by pulling your navel toward your spine. Hold this position for a few seconds. It's useful for strengthening the deep core muscles and improving posture.

9

Let's Be Real

L et's be real. Some of us cannot afford to tackle our weight issues on our own. There are many WHY's behind the scenes.

Did you know that some people gain or lose weight when they grieve? We may need to visit our doctors, nutritionists, therapists, and specialists to determine where to start.

Yes, they might find something. Yes, they are likely to say something that we already know and don't want confirmed. Yes, we may have to revisit old wounds and hurts that are neatly buried. Still, we have to choose to face our hang ups and make the necessary changes.

We cannot conquer our weight goals, when our stress, low self esteem, bitterness, procrastination, fear, perfectionism, anxiety, depression, and the like have deep root systems that are preventing us from moving forward. We must confront our trauma(s) and be willing to seek help.

It's time to acknowledge and address that not all weight issues are related to food. Let's deal with our stuff and truly overcome our hindrances and shortcomings to become all that we're designed to be.

10

Results

We know that we are moving "enough" when we are not graduating upwards in pants and dress sizes. We know it when our clothes fit comfortably and our bodies feel strong and energized. Another way to measure progress can be a specific number on the scale, but it doesn't have to be that way. It's okay to measure progress in different ways.

11

Conclusion

So, long story short, there are several ways to make fitness a part of your daily life. This guide leaves no excuses for not fitting movement into every day. Choose ways that work for you and be consistent with them. Make it a priority by scheduling it, doing it with friends, or by incorporating it into your daily tasks and pleasures. Develop consistency in your sleep schedule and seek guidance from practitioners and other professionals as needed. If desired, use an app or go to the gym. Take action to determine the direction of your life and position yourself to live a fulfilling and high-quality life.

Remember that consistency is key when it comes to daily fitness. Enjoy your life journey towards a healthier and happier you!

Call to action

Take some time today to pick 2 or more daily fitness habits that you can begin to apply immediately. Experiment with the others as you see fit.

If you found this book helpful, I would greatly appreciate it if you could tell 3 friends or family members about it and leave a positive review on Amazon!

12

Resources

OpenAI. (2024). ChatGPT (GPT-4) [Software]. OpenAI. https://www.openai.com/chatgpt

Noom, Inc. (n.d.). About Noom. Retrieved June 17, 2024, from https://www.noom.com/

Noom. (2024). In Wikipedia. Retrieved June 17, 2024, from https://en.wikipedia.org/wiki/Noom

JustFit. (2024). At home workouts for women, female fitness quotes. Retrieved from https://justfit.app/

ViralTalky. (2024). JustFit app review: Is it worth the hype? Retrieved June 17, 2024, from https://viraltalky.com/justfit-app-review/